EMOTIONALLY MANAGING YOUR ILLNESS

Dr. Talya Miron-Shatz and the Buddy&Soul team

INTRODUCTION: WELCOME TO EMOTIONALLY MANAGING YOUR ILLNESS

Being ill is not easy. A lot is going on, and very little of it is fun. Being asked "how are you feeling?" might be nice the first few thousand times, but eventually it seems either redundant (I feel terrible! Still! But thanks for asking…) or like a sham (I'm falling apart at the seams, but I'll beam a smile and say "fine" because I don't have the energy to entertain pity). It may also seem beside the point, because you are ill, physically unwell, so what else is there to know? But, connecting with how you feel is actually one of the most important parts of having and managing a disease. When we're ill, we may sometimes forget to stop and take our own pulse, and ask, how am I feeling? What is going on with me?

This is important because it helps us remember who we were before we were 'a patient' and that's the unspoken part of being unwell. It may strip your other identities, erode them, and leave you scared, confused, angry, lost, and in pain. But inside, you know that's not the real you or at least, not the only real you.

For most of my career as a researcher, I have chosen to focus on medical decision making, feeling that the one thing I can do to make the world a better place, if only marginally. This is what this course is also trying to do – to make your world a (even marginally) better place.

Obviously, emotionally managing your illness won't magically make you better. It won't make the disease disappear, the maladies subside, or the doctors wrong. But that's not the aim. The doctors have the best chance at helping your body, but only you can sort things out emotionally, and find your own strength to best play the (crappy) hand you've been dealt. The illness didn't just happen; it happened to a person, it happened to you. And the feelings you're dealing with right now may not be logged in your electronic health record and may not receive as much attention as your physical symptoms, but they really do matter.

There are three goals that we had in mind while creating this book. We want you to:

- Identify, map out and sort your feelings regarding your illness.
- Find strength and emotional balance to see you through your medical condition.
- Take responsibility for your emotional well-being during your illness.

When you're dealing with illness you may feel like your life is unbalanced, like you're taking a sharp turn too fast, or trying to run a marathon without the proper training or gear. This course will help you get your emotions in check, or at least understand what you're feeling, so that you are better able to deal with everything that's going on.

YOUR JOURNEY TO EMOTIONALLY MANAGING YOUR ILLNESS

HOW TO USE THIS BOOK TO EMOTIONALLY MANAGE YOUR ILLNESS

In this book you'll find ten great strategies for achieving the goals we listed above. You'll also find inspiring content and exercises you can engage with to help you practice emotionally managing your illness.

You will get the most out of this book by going through the strategies and associated exercises one by one. Of course, you can also simply read it the whole way through. But we recommend using this book by going through it in order, watching the TED talks, and doing the exercises. We have found the best way to do the exercises is by dedicating a notebook as your course journal. If you're reading this book on a PC, feel free to create a text file and use that as your course journal. Or you could simply use a good ol' pen and paper to do the exercises. Either way, we recommend keeping some method of writing handy while you go through the exercises in this book to optimize what you get out of it.

To maximize your experience with the Buddy and Soul book, share your thoughts and insights with us on social media! Post pictures relating to your progress on Instagram and Twitter, tagging @Buddy_N_Soul, and Facebook @Buddy&Soul.   By sharing with us on social media, not only can you help others with their personal journeys, you can read about those facing similar challenges.

Direct message us YOUR story @Buddy_N_Soul on Instagram and be anonymously featured for a chance to **win a Buddy&Soul three month free membership**.

If you really want to go all the way, visit our website, BuddynSoul.com, and explore all that we have to offer beyond 'Emotionally Managing your Illness'. In fact, we have two other books in the Medical Series that we think you might benefit from: Manage Your Medical Condition and Adhering to Your Medication

WHY I CREATED BUDDY&SOUL AND WHY I CREATED THIS BOOK.

I'm Dr. Talya Miron-Shatz, CEO of Buddy&Soul, where Emotionally Managing Your Illness and many more e-courses and books come from. I have a PhD in psychology and was very fortunate to do my post-doc at Princeton University with Nobel Laureate Daniel Kahneman. I've also taught at the Wharton Business School, University of Pennsylvania. Now I'm a professor at the Ono Academic College, and a visiting researcher at Cambridge University. I used to study happiness, and for a long time now, I've been studying medical decision making and helping organizations support people on their way to joy and health. One thing that struck me as unfair was that we were expecting people to change their life

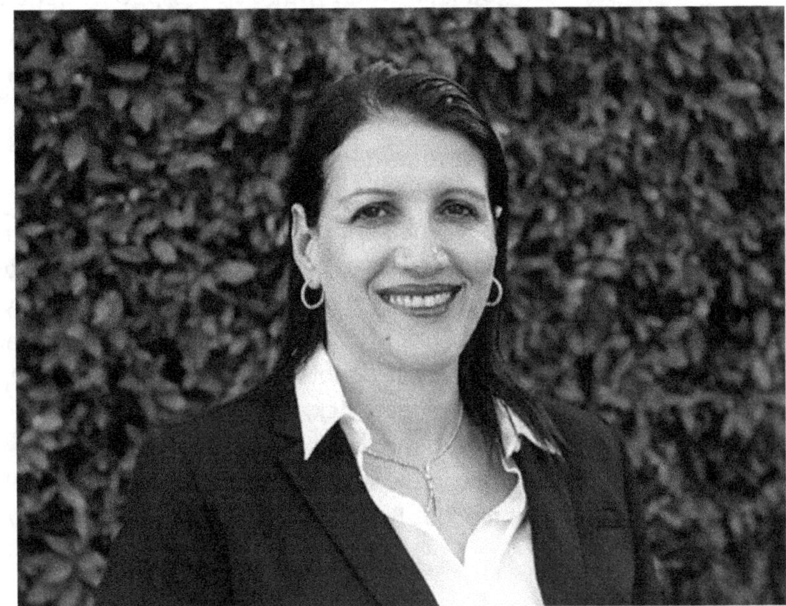

for good but weren't giving them the tools to do so. People deserve all the help they can get when breaking out of old patterns and moving their lives forward.

This is what Buddy&Soul does.

We support you in many ways by providing science-based actionable ways to sustain your body and mind. We help you sleep better, spark a change in your eating habits, and manage stress. We teach you how to create new habits and how to engage your willpower. We help you grow, claim your self-esteem, cultivate authenticity, reframe your life story, achieve your goals and so much more. Including Emotionally Manage Your Illness.

Everything you need to change your life for good.

I want to hear from YOU! Please feel free to send me an email with your thoughts, suggestions, and feedback regarding this book to talya@buddynsoul.com. I would love to hear what you think about this book and how it helped you with emotionally managing your illness. Your feedback is extremely valuable and will allow us to help more individuals, like yourself, to obtain the necessary tools and support needed to change their lives for good.

10 Reasons to emotionally manage your illness

There's so much going on when you're sick. Appointments, treatments, exercise, and diet. In the hectic day-to-day, you need to take control of your emotions, not just the practical stuff. Here's why.

1. Practicing this course will help you sort out your feelings, which can feel like a huge load off your mind.
2. It's important to remember to make an emotional check of yourself, not just a physical check. Your emotions are part of the disease, too.
3. This course will help you find the positive even in the negative. Oh, and it also reminds you that sometimes you need to give those negative emotions some space, they're important too.
4. This course will give you tips and tricks to keeping yourself emotionally balanced. An illness needs lots of care, after all, even if it's just maintenance.
5. Living with illness is doable, but you can also *thrive.*
6. When your body gets sick, so do your emotions. You need to heal not only on a physical level, but on an emotional level as well.
7. Emotions play an essential role in managing your illness; ignoring them might not make your things worse, but it will keep you from feeling truly *well.*

Add your own:

8. ____

9. ____

10. ____

Should you even continue to emotionally manage your illness?

With all the craziness that is your life right now due to your medical condition, is now really the right time to be emotionally managing your illness? Is personal growth and development a luxury for the healthy, or can you too benefit from finding emotional balance amongst the upheaval?

For:

1. It is precisely because of your illness that you should be emotionally managing your illness.
2. When's *not* a good time to benefit from emotional balance?
3. Happiness is known to benefit a person both emotionally and physically.
4. What, now that you're sick, you give up on your own movement and growth?

Add your own argument:

5. ____

Against:

1. I'm much too frail to take on added pressures, like emotionally managing my illness.
2. How many times do I need to say this? My emotions are fine! It's my body that's sick.
3. Managing emotions is for healthy people.
4. I want to be emotionally unstable! It's part of being sick.

Add your own argument:

5. ____

My turning point with emotionally managing my illness

Were you also resistant to the very idea of emotionally managing an illness, let alone to practicing it? What was your turning point, and how did it play out? Take a few moments to write about this experience in your journal, and then share your story with the Buddy and Soul community!

Direct message us YOUR story @Buddy_N_Soul on Instagram and be anonymously featured for a chance to **win a Buddy&Soul three month free membership**.

Strategy 1: Take Your Internal Pulse

Being ill puts a heavy emphasis on your body – but what about your mind? Surely your mind is not quite at peace at this moment either. While doctors and nurses are taking your pulse, analyzing your blood, tapping your knees for reflexes, and shining a light into your pupils, chances are no one is taking your internal pulse, checking in on how you are feeling, on all levels. In case you're wondering why it matters at a time when body should be in the center, let me explain. According to Triune Brain Theory, your brain is made up of three parts – the neocortex (your thinking brain), the limbic system (your feeling brain), and your brain stem (your reptilian/gut instinct brain). If your body is in stress, then that influences all three parts of your brain. Your illness is not isolated to the body; it has an impact on all three levels.

Checking in with your internal pulse to become aware of your thoughts, feelings, and gut instincts is a crucial piece of battling your illness. And this isn't me arguing this; it's Professor Daniel J Siegel, a UCLA-based clinical psychiatrist, in his book *Mindsight* (p. 14-22).

These three parts, which include your willpower, your resilience, and your joie de vivre, will help carry you through these trying times. **Even if connecting with yourself internally cannot help you get physically better, it can help you be happier and more at peace about your condition.**

Additionally, sometimes we'll turn all our mental acumen inwards to determine that we feel… nothing. But even so, we should stop and ask whether this *nothing* is a form of acceptance, or a rushed lid we slammed down on anxiety, anger, denial, or a combination of all three. Whatever you're feeling about your illness – well, that's just how you feel. There's no judging. But, if you recognize your emotions, and deal with them, you could be at a better place.

EXERCISE

Take your internal pulse right now. The next few minutes are for you to relax and focus on *you*, so go ahead and get in the right headspace. Take some deep breaths and then, in your journal, write out how you feel about your condition.

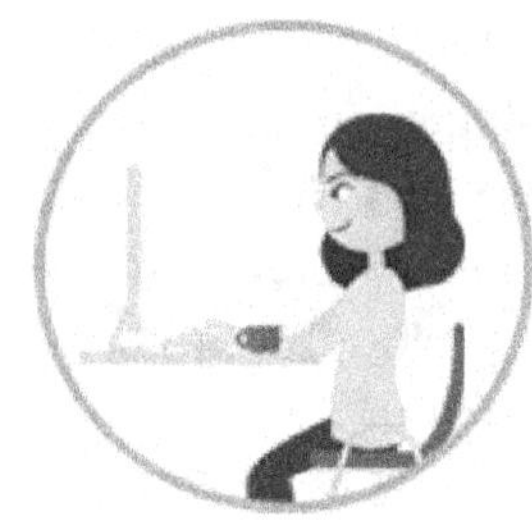

You can list anything from, "I'm not involved as I'd like to be" to "I wish I could just hide under the covers and have someone sort it out for me" to "I could really listen to my gut more." This list is entirely for you.

Then use your journal to write a validating note to yourself that whatever you're thinking and feeling is normal and okay.

TIPS

Tip 1: If you feel your thoughts wandering, don't judge them. Gently bring yourself back to the question of your illness and how you feel about it.

Tip 2: If you feel at a loss, imagine you were talking it out with someone you are open and honest with – a spouse, a parent, a close friend, or maybe a random stranger sitting next to you on a long train ride whom you will never meet again.

Tip 3: According to a study, it's been proven that goal-setting is an effective way to support self-help behaviors. You can use this for reference and extra motivation as you continue to work through the rest of this course.

(Plus, check out our Achieve Your Goals course 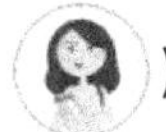)

Tip 4: Remember this is about discovering what you're feeling and validating anything that needs a head nod. This is the first step to tackling anything negative that may be holding you back for successful emotional management.

Tip 5: Are your stress symptoms impacting your health? Check out our Stress Management course. 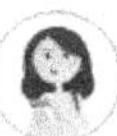

DRIVING THE MESSAGE HOME

I'm glad that you've decided to join us for the course Emotionally Manage Your Illness. Each session of our course consists of a warm-up talk followed by a hands-on component where you'll learn a new skill or idea and have a chance to start putting it into action.

We're going to start the Emotionally Manage Your Illness course by taking a fundamental look at taking your internal pulse.

In this innovative TED Talk, Guy Winch introduces us to a new concept: emotional hygiene. We'll go to the doctor when we feel flu-ish or a nagging pain. So why don't we see a health professional when we feel emotional pain: guilt, loss, loneliness? Too many of us deal with common psychological-health issues on our own, says Winch. But we don't have to. He makes a compelling case to practice emotional hygiene — taking care of our emotions, our minds, with the same diligence we take care of our bodies.

So let's begin to bridge the gap between physical health and emotional health because both can harm your wellbeing. Let's up our emotional hygiene and take our internal pulse. Let's really start to understand what's going on with us.

We think you'll find that the more you put into the course, the more you'll get out of it. So take full advantage of all our features and find your place in a community of people facing similar challenges.

Watch 'How to Practice Emotional First Aid' presented by Guy Winch on YouTube.

9 Emotions that affect how you manage illness

Your mood affects the way you think, the way you feel, and how you emotionally manage your disease. Here are some emotions you may be experiencing and how they may be impacting you.

(Plus: Check out our Declutter Your Mind course 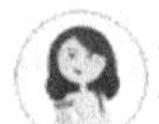)

1. **Anger.** When your blood is boiling, wanting to overflow, you can't help but feel edgy around everybody, from your loved ones to medical personnel. Anger is an emotion that gets the body ready to fight. So let's experience the anger, and then try to tone it down. Your body needs to store its energy to fight more important things, like the disease.
2. **Shame.** This little embarrassed voice of self-blame is ringing in your ears, making you feel responsible and ashamed of being ill. Know that you are not to blame for your illness. You did nothing wrong, and you deserve the help you need to get through this.
3. **Sadness.** Are you experiencing a sense of mourning for your old and healthy self? A need to cry? Well, let the tears happen. Allowing them to flow freely will release some of the tension your body is experiencing from being sick.
4. **Happiness.** Although a contrast to the previous emotions, being sick also helps heighten your positive feelings such as happiness. A new appreciation for the little gifts in life is born.
5. **Hopefulness.** Sometimes it takes something like illness to help us redefine our lives and priorities. With this newfound direction and hope, we can feel like a totally new human being.
6. **Calmness.** This incredible feeling that comes when you feel at one with the moment. Even with illness.

Did we miss anything? Add it in your journal:

7. ____

8. ____

9. ____

My illness is all physical – forget the "internal pulse."

When we go to the doctor for a check-up, the doctor checks our bodies, and ignores the rest of us. So when the body gets sick, *we* also tend to forget about the greater us. That's where checking your 'internal pulse' comes in.

For:

1. My body is sick. So what? The rest of me is feeling fine.
2. Illness is by definition a physical thing. My mental well-being can never get 'sick.'
3. Sometimes I do feel not well. Right now I'm totally fine. Stop trying to push problems where there are none.
4. So what if I don't feel great – the focus is on my physical illness, not my emotional state. When my body gets well, also my mood will get better.
5. My feelings don't influence my physical well-being.

Add your own argument:

6. ____

Against:

1. My emotional world greatly influences my body and how I'm feeling. If I'm feeling happy and full, then my illness doesn't impact me the same way.
2. It's all about the mind-body connection nowadays.
3. Think good be good, no?
4. I wouldn't be true to me if I didn't take care of my internal world in addition to my disease.
5. I pretend I'm handling everything, but inside, I'm scared and worried and scared, again. This is not being emotionally well.

Add your own argument:

6. ____

How taking my "internal pulse" helped me manage my illness

A big chunk of life is led on autopilot, and this becomes all the more true when managing an illness. You go into survival mode and sometimes even you forget that there's a person in there, and not just an illness. Share how stopping to take your internal pulse helped you take a minute to reflect, and to manage your illness.

Take some time brainstorming in your journal about your experience with managing your illness, and then share your story with the Buddy and Soul community! Tag us on Instagram and Twitter @Buddy_N_Soul, using the **#BuddynSoulMedSupport**. By sharing with us on social media, not only can you help others with their personal journeys, you can read about those facing similar challenges.

Call me a skeptic, but 'emotional hygiene'? for illness? please.

In Guy Winch's TED Talk, *Why we all need to practice emotional first aid,* Winch discusses the importance of emotional hygiene; similar to going to a doctor when we're physically not well, we need to be equally concerned with our emotional well-being. But seriously… seriously?

For:

1. I'm offended by the comparison. Physical ailments make you sick, but emotional ones? They only make you moody.
2. How can you measure something like emotional hygiene? Unlike germs, you can't see sadness under a microscope and it's not like someone else can look at you and know what you're feeling.
3. I've heard a lot of alternative theories for coping with illness, but this really takes the cake.

Add your own argument:

4. ____

Against:

1. I'm not sure why the idea of 'emotional hygiene' comes with so much skepticism. Mental health professionals do exactly that: diagnose feelings.
2. I'm into the whole mind-body package. If your mind (i.e. your emotions) are not well, that influences your physical health, and vice versa.
   (Plus: Check out our Mindfulness for Beginners course)
3. When I feel blue, it influences my energy level and my daily function. I can only imagine that if my feelings were more intensified, then my energy level and daily functioning would only be further impacted.

Add your own argument:

4. ____

Strategy 2: Define your disease "rough spots"

Does it help to commiserate? Let's give it a try.

A comprehensive study spanning over 8,000 patients from 17 countries affirmed what we already reported, and what you may know first-hand: illness affects much more than your body. Forty percent of patients reported that medication was interfering with their way of life. But this is an obvious area where an illness would interfere. Other areas, such as social, sexual or emotional can be more surprising, which illustrates how widely and deeply living with a disease can paint your life.

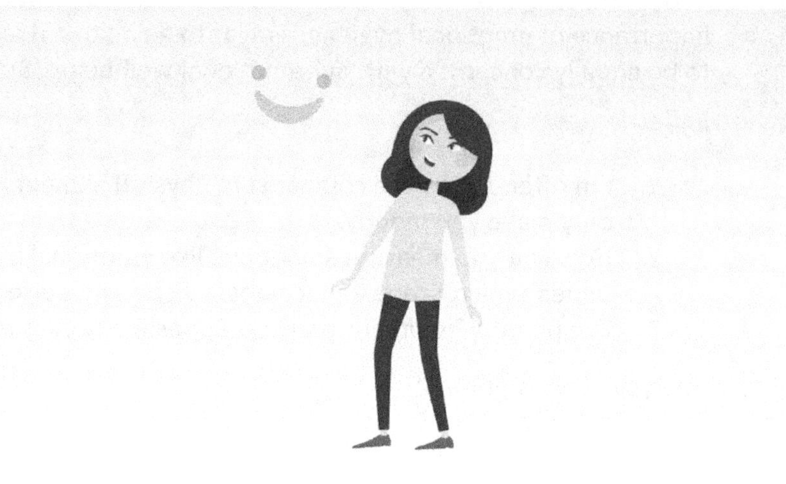

What I mean by commiserating is taking a moment to **point out to yourself, honestly, what effects this illness has had on your life, letting these effects sink in, and then congratulating yourself on dealing with it for however long you've been dealing with it.**

For one, I feel that realizing that others share your challenges and maybe the difficulties you're encountering and that can be a huge relief. It's not that you're doing anything wrong. It's that it's difficult. For everyone.

In this day and age, when we're constantly probed to think positive, and believe in the healing power of our thoughts, feeling bad is almost obscene. But let's do it anyway.

Why? Because if you identify, for example, that financial issues around your medical condition are bothering you, it'll be a good cue to take care of them. Not just for money's sake, but for your mental well-being.

If it's any comfort, in this study, no one country's outcomes were consistently better or worse than others.

EXERCISE

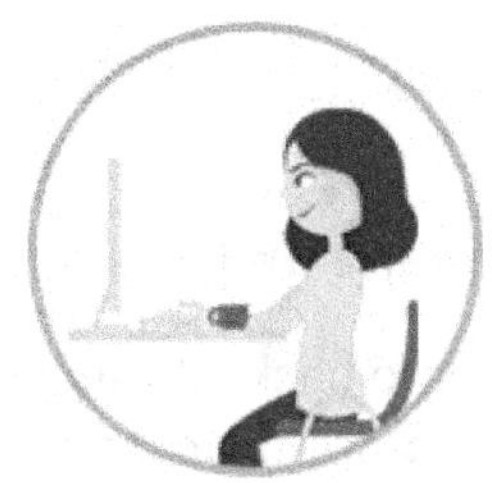

Step 1: **Take this survey to determine your concerns regarding your medical condition.** (These are most people's prime concerns, according to a large-scale study.)

What are your primary illness upsets?

1. Physical health
2. Financial concerns
3. Just tired of always dealing with it
4. Influences work or studies
5. Messes with my leisure activities
6. Relationships with friends/family

Step 2:

Write yourself a fan letter filled with praise. Focus on what you've experienced the most success with in your medical journey and congratulate yourself for dealing it with it as long as you have and as well as you have. Yes, even if you moaned about it.

TIP

Tip 1: Remember, it's an objectively tough reality you're living in, and you deserve to receive heartfelt kudos for tackling it.

DRIVING THE MESSAGE HOME

Why aren't we more compassionate?

Welcome back. In this TED Talk, Daniel Goleman, author of *Emotional Intelligence*, asks why we aren't more compassionate more of the time. On one hand, we'd like to think that compassion for others is intuitive. Why wouldn't our friends and family know exactly what it is we need all the time? On the other hand, there is so much going on in our own lives that seeing the needs of others is overshadowed by our own needs.

The research seems to demonstrate that unless we are consciously tuning in to the needs of others, our default setting is to focus on our own needs. With this in mind, the best way to get the compassion we need is to ask for it. And, the best way to get the help we want is to request it.

Watch 'Why Aren't We All Good Samaritans?' presented by Daniel Goleman on YouTube.

Disease sucks. Can't I just leave it at that?

Break it down; know what bothers you, exactly… But why bother? It won't change how much I'm bothered; it will only give me a different name to call it. I just don't see the point.

For:

1. I just don't see how the breakdown matters. The situation as a whole just sucks.

2. Each individual thing is manageable; it's the culmination of it all that's really rotten for me.

3. Breaking down my "rough-spots" into specifics feels somehow like it's lessening my right to feel how hard it's been.

Add your own argument:

4. ____

Against:

1. When I break it down, it helps me realize what's really been troubling me, and what's just been a nuisance.

2. I'm the type of person who needs to call things as they are. "Sucks" is just too broad a term for me to tackle effectively.

3. For me, when I find a specific rough-spot, it allows me to really feel sorry for myself, for that specific thing, for as long as I need to, rather than gloss it over as general suckage.

Add your own argument:

4 ____

9 Annoying life side effects of illness

Coping with an illness can come with a bucket-load of physical and emotional side effects—some of which will never appear in the medical literature. These types of side-effects may be left unspoken, but boy, are they hard to live with. Here are some that really take the cake:

1. "Let's all go to lunch!" … The words ring out, and can make you cringe. Unfortunately, not many people are taking into consideration all the dietary restrictions of your illness.

2. Some friends are planning a trip abroad and would love for you to join them! They just have to check their passport is valid, and you have to make sure you're allowed to travel with your meds, figure out medical centers wherever you go, and extend your travel insurance 7 ways from Sunday.

3. "Oh, but you don't *look* sick." Somehow this makes you feel like a hypochondriac exaggerating an illness, just because *they* can't see it.

4. "Come out with us tonight, we *never* see you!" Sometimes, you really can't go out, and nobody seems to understand it's not personal, it's just been a tiring day.

5. "I'm sorry you're not feeling well. I've also been under the weather lately." Other's well-meaning empathy doesn't seem to cut it on the tough days.

6. "Maybe you should get out of the house. You'd feel better." You want to be as active as those around you, but some days it can take so much energy just to get out of bed.

Add your own:

7. ____

8. ____

9. ____

The illness "rough spots" I nipped in the bud

You could see them coming a mile away, and you plotted a new course to avoid them as best as you could. These are the rough spots you were able to nip in the bud! Share your story with the community, and help inspire others to be pro-active with their illness rough spots.

Take some time brainstorming in your journal about your experience with managing your illness, and then share your story with the Buddy and Soul community! Direct message us YOUR story @Buddy_N_Soul on Instagram and be anonymously featured for a chance to **win a Buddy&Soul three month free membership**. You can also tag us on Instagram and Twitter @Buddy_N_Soul, using the **#BuddynSoulMedSupport**. By sharing with us on social media, not only can you help others with their personal journeys, you can read about those facing similar challenges.

Whose support do you value when you're sick?

Being sick is a big challenge. Not only is your body ill, but your emotions are out of sync as well. Who is your go-to person when you need some help emotionally managing your illness?

1. I prefer to work through my illness alone
2. My partner
3. My children
4. Family and friends
5. My healthcare team

Did we miss anything? Add it in your journal:

6. ____

7. ____

8. ____

Strategy 3: Get all the help you can

When ill, you naturally seek medical help but that may not be all the help you need, especially as illness affects your entire life. You might need also psychological, emotional, spiritual, and even financial help. Many of us feel we can brave everything on our own, or at least that we should be able to. But when we are sick, we need support from others. This does not mean we are weak or incapable. It only means we need people who will help us work through difficult times.

It's a bit of a vicious cycle, since the harsher the disease, the more help we will probably need, and yet the more difficult it often becomes to ask for that help.

There are so many assumptions that are made about asking for help. And usually, many are simply not true. For example, I always worry that if I ask for help I have to be ready and willing to reciprocate. My sister once told me she hates asking for help because she doesn't want to seem like a burden. And I know my perfectionist best friend never asks for help because he's convinced nobody can ever do things as well as he himself can do them. When I checked in with others about these assumptions, I was surprised to learn they were not true. My family and friends wanted to help me, they were simply waiting for me to take that first step and ask.

Building on what you identified last session as your main concerns, today you'll be translating your needs into ways to get help.

Frank Flynn, associate professor of organizational behavior at Stanford Graduate School of Business, says that we shouldn't assume that others are disinclined to help us. "People are more willing to help than you think, and that can be important to know when you're trying to get the resources you need to get a job done, when you're trying to solicit funds, or what have you" (Rigoglioso, 2008).

Ask yourself, if the tables were turned, how would you feel if a friend asked you for help? Or how happy would it make you knowing that your sick friend got psychological help when she needed it? What about financial support? If you had the money, would you not be glad to give it to a friend in need? Now flip the tables back. Just as you would be happy to support a friend or family member in need, and just as you would not view their request for help in a demeaning way, think of yourself in the same manner.

EXERCISE

In your journal, **list the areas where you could use some help and support around managing your illness.** If this seems overwhelming, try to think of the smallest thing that could make you feel better.

Does it involve someone making you cheesecake? You know, just to reward you for bravely swallowing that medication that makes you cringe. Driving you from treatments? Folding your laundry? Or giving you a mushy, marshmallow hug?

Then, **create a caring 'wish list'** where you write down the names of people or institutions that could potentially help you with each task: think family members, friends, clergy, members of your community, co-workers, professionals, community organizations, or acquaintances who have gone through similar experiences.

TIPS

Tip 1: Make this happen: choose one person or help avenue from your list and contact them today, or schedule it in your calendar. Do not be shy. Chances are you'll at *least* be well received. I'm betting the person on the other side will surprise you.

Tip 2: If you feel bad about asking for help, ask yourself – would I give the kind of help I am asking for? If the answer is 'yes!' go ahead and ask for it. It is not a weakness to ask for assistance – if anything it's a sign of strength.

Tip 3: People are always asking 'what can I do for you,' or 'can I do anything to help?' Now you know what to say!

Tip 4: Asking for help may be a skill we need to acquire and develop, so now's the perfect opportunity to start.

Tip 5: Support means different things to everyone. When you imagine support, think of the type of help that you'd really truly like to receive, but possibly don't dare ask for. Sometimes, even in our minds we don't dare go to that place where we have to let down our guard and actually rely on someone else.

Tip 6: Are you uncertain what help you really need? Check out our Cultivating Authenticity course. 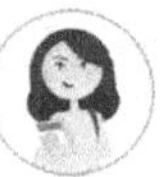

DRIVING THE MESSAGE HOME

According to organizational psychologist Adam Grant, there are three types of people: givers, takers, and matchers (who keep an even balance between giving and taking). Are you curious which type of person succeeds the most? And how that can influence whether or not you ask for help when you need it? Well enjoy the following TED Talk to find out! Remember to keep in mind that when someone takes, they provide the opportunity for someone else to give, and vice versa. Enjoy!

(Plus: Check out our Defining Your Identity course 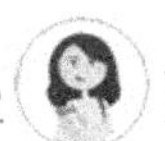)

Watch 'Are You a Giver or a Taker' presented Adam Grant on YouTube.

What's holding you back from asking for help?

Emotionally and physically managing our illness alone is almost impossible. And yet, it's so hard sometimes to ask for help! What keeps you from getting the help you deserve?

1. Asking for help is a sign of weakness.
2. Asking for help means I'm losing control of the situation.
3. Asking for help means I need to reciprocate that help, and right now I'm not able to do that.
4. Asking for help makes me a burden.
5. Asking for help is pointless because only I can get it right.

Did we miss anything? Add it in your journal:

6. ____

Emotionally managing an illness means NOT asking for help.

As an adult, you've always been independent and self-sufficient. Now that you're ill, you're wondering: Should you ask for help? Or will that be the final straw that breaks your competent sense of self? (Plus: Check out our Defining Your Identity course)

For:

1. You are independent and only you know what's best for you!
2. You've dealt with many challenges in your life before this one and have managed to survive on your own. How is this any different?
3. Just like too many cooks spoil the broth, too many people involved in your medical process may overwhelm you and complicate your experience unnecessarily.
4. Why should you burden your family members, who have their own problems, with your disease?
5. If you manage your disease alone then sometimes you can try to pretend it doesn't exist.
6. People will pity you and act differently towards you if they know you are sick.
7. Every patient is unique. Being in the same boat as others does not help me.
8. I often find that a group is overpowered by one loud person, and then nobody listens to me. Might as well proceed alone.

Add your own argument:

9. ____

Against:

1. Dealing with disease often prevents you from dealing with other aspects of your life. If you allow others to be involved, then you'll be ensuring that your dog is being fed and your flowers are being watered.
2. Managing disease by yourself can make you feel isolated and lonely, while sharing the burden takes some of the load off you. Aren't you dealing with enough as is?
3. It is always important to get a second opinion - and it's as true on the emotional front as it is on the medical front! Checking in with people who care about you can help you streamline your emotions and keep them balanced.
4. Your emotional well-being contributes to your physical well-being. Studies show that sharing your experiences and talking about your illness with the right people can improve your emotional health.
5. If you're going to beat this disease, you need the whole team to be fighting along with you!

Add your own argument:

6. ____

Asking for help eased the 'being sick' burden

Asking for help comes easily for some people, but for others it's a burden in its own right. But sometimes taking that plunge can have benefits unforeseen. Read on to see how members of the community found the courage to ask for help, and how it ultimately helped them in new ways.

3 Insights about giving from Grant's talk

According to Adam Grant's TED Talk *Are you a giver or a taker,* the way to success is through giving. Here are some great ways to initiate giving both personally and socially.

1. Keep the giving small so you don't burn out.
2. Be sure to leave time for your own responsibilities amongst the giving.
3. Promote asking; there is more giving when someone asks for help.

Strategy 4: Keep tabs on your feelings

For some people, finding a way to express themselves
to others is simply too much of an obstacle to
overcome... Which is fine. To others, speaking about
their emotions is second nature. But this can change
when life deals an uncomfortable hand.

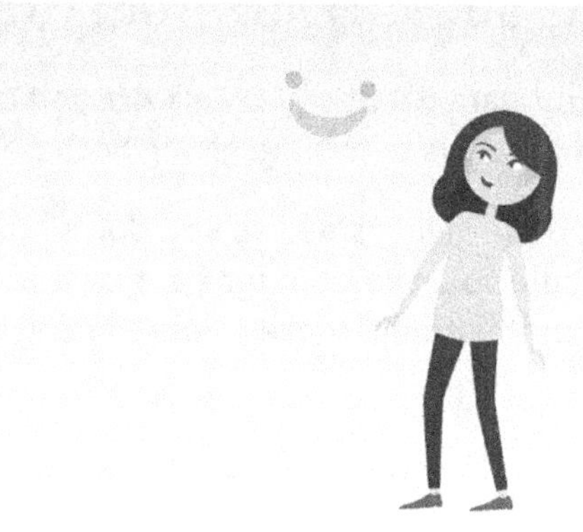

When facing an illness, you don't need to add things to
your plate that will cause more stress. However,
expressing yourself throughout your illness is beneficial
for your mental wellbeing. It allows you to identify and
work through your feelings — even the ones you're not so proud of. It's a much better way to live than
keeping your emotions bottled up, being embarrassed, or feeling isolated because no one really knows
how you feel. And if you don't want to or can't talk – write!

I know. "Dear Diary, today I had blood work," or, "Just got back from the hospital. Worst part was I
couldn't remember where I parked my car, I was in such a hurry this morning" don't exactly seem like
the kinds of things you want to save for posterity. But, posterity be damned, keeping a journal, or
another form of expression, can help you work towards several important ends. It can help you figure
out how you're feeling, what is making things great for you, and what – not so much. The science has
repeatedly demonstrated the importance for those struggling with illness to find an outlet for emotional
expression:

1. A study of women with early-stage breast cancer were asked to write their deepest thoughts
    and feelings over a four-session span. Results showed that the women who journaled reported
    significantly decreased medical symptoms and fewer medical appointments.
2. A study of patients with varying stages of renal cell carcinoma (RCC) demonstrated that those
    who wrote about their feelings toward their cancer reported reduced cancer-related symptoms
    and improved physical functioning.
3. In a study of adult leukemia and lymphoma patients, participants were asked to complete a 20-
    minute writing session while waiting for an appointment followed by a post-writing assignment
    and a follow-up journaling session three weeks later. Results showed that even after one writing
    session, the way patients thought about their medical condition changed. As a result, they also
    reported better quality of life after journaling about their illness.

Here's how it's done: You need to keep track of some basic info every day. You can do it in your
Buddy&Soul journal, or use a journal app or an honest-to-God paper-and-binding notebook. Find which
option works best for you and encourages you to keep journaling. A journal and careful logging can
assign meaning to your medical condition. It can help you note changes and connections between
phenomena that you wouldn't have thought about otherwise. It can help you remember the good times,
and also the bad times, and how you overcame them. And it can help you transform the illness-related
events in your life into anecdotes and help put them behind you. Last but not least, a journal can be a
place where you pour your heart out and talk about all the things you don't want to share with anybody,
but need to get out of your system nonetheless.

A journal can be about anything you like. As long as you're connecting with yourself to write it.

So let's get to it!

EXERCISE

Try a bite-sized version and **write your very first journal entry.** It doesn't have to be anything fancy. Jot down whatever thoughts and feelings come to mind. If you're not sure where to start, try – 'this is how my medical condition affected my day' and 'this is how it made me feel'.

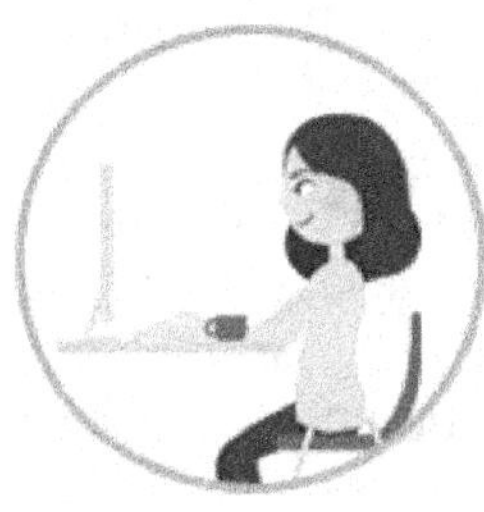

TIPS

Tip 1: Not the journaling type? Still, try it, just this once. You might be surprised.

Tip 2: You can start small and be laconic. Writing may grow on you.

Tip 3: At a loss for words? Upload a photo instead. This is the beginning of your journaling journey!

Tip 4: Scrapbooking is a fun way to journal if you enjoy an artistic challenge.

Tip 5: You can keep use the same journal that you use for this course and come every day just to add a line or two about your ups and downs and general mood or feelings.

Tip 6: If you want to make journaling a top priority or daily habit and are struggling, be sure to check out our Priorities Reboot and Habit Workshop courses.

DRIVING THE MESSAGE HOME

Despite the unfortunate "cards he was dealt," Julmar Carcedo, an international student on financial aid from Davao, Philippines, managed to find happiness on Brown's campus. In this TEDx Talk, he shares his personal journey and gives us advice on finding our happiness through journaling, a key outlet for emotional expression during times of illness and health. From a place of anger and hurt, Carcedo was able to transform his life into one of happiness and hope. He offers several helpful tips for journaling that can help you if you decide to try your own form of journaling throughout your illness.

Watch 'Journal Your Way to Happiness' presented by Julmar Carcedo at TEDxBrownU on YouTube.

10 Journaling tips to help you emotionally manage your illness

Even if you're not the journaling type, when you're ill a journal can be a great outlet for your emotions. Here are a few tips to get you started.

1. Decide on format – will you use a journal, a computer, your Buddy&Soul journal, or a mobile app? This is especially important if you're unused to journaling in the first place. You need to find a medium you feel comfortable with that will encourage you to continue even when things get tough.

2. Make a habit of it. There will be days when the last thing you want to do is sit down and write, and on these days you'll need the power of habit to carry you through.
    (Plus: Check out our Habit Workshop course)

3. Date each entry. You may think you'll remember when an event occurred, because the memory is so powerful, but our minds tend to forget. Looking back on these entries, you'll want to know when your feelings changed, or what precipitated a major reaction.

4. If you can't seem to think of what to write, just jot down the date and technical things that happened on the day: whom you met with or spoke to, what you had for breakfast. Don't pressure yourself to only write the "important" things.

5. Try playing relaxing music or setting a relaxing mood when writing. Pretend you're an 18th Century novelist if it gets your writing going.

6. Suspend judgment. Write whatever comes to mind. No one's reading your journal but you!

7. Try to dream of the future you want for yourself, sans illness. Write it out.
    (Plus: Check out our Achieve Your Goals course)

Do you have any tips? Add your own!

8. ____

9. ____

10. ____

What could inspire you to write about your illness?

There are so many things we can do to help us emotionally manage our illness, one of them being journaling. And yet, when it comes down to writing about illness, there's a roadblock. What would help inspire you to take the next step and journal about your illness?

1. Accessibility. The ability to turn to my journal whenever and wherever I want.
2. The sheer sense of accomplishment that comes with actually following through on   something.
3. Believing that journaling and expressing is good for my mental and physical well-being.
4. Doing something! Journaling helps me feel less helpless!
5. Nothing. Journaling is not inspiring for me.

List your own:

6. ____

7. ____

8. ____

How channeling my anger helped my illness

Anger at being ill is normal, and even a good sign. But there's a balance to be struck between feeling it, and letting it overpower you. Have you found that balance? Share with the community how you channeled your anger in a way that helped you manage your illness.

Take some time brainstorming in your journal about your experience with managing your illness, and then share your story with the Buddy and Soul community! Tag us on Instagram and Twitter @Buddy_N_Soul, using the **#BuddynSoulMedSupport**. You can also direct message us YOUR story @Buddy_N_Soul on Instagram and be anonymously featured for a chance to **win a Buddy&Soul three month free membership**. By sharing with us on social media, not only can you help others with their personal journeys, you can read about those facing similar challenges.

My journal turned my illness experience around...Here's how

I was skeptical about the concept of journaling, but in the end, it taught me more than I thought it could. Here is how keeping a journal helped me emotionally manage my medical condition. Hopefully this can help inspire others to share their journaling experiences, too.

Strategy 5: Make time to mope

We're often taught that we have two options: Either be perceived as weak or show that stiff upper-lip. Be a needy coward or face up to life's challenges. Fuss, or *do something* about it.

When we're kids, this means to always be the bigger person, always share, never whine, and soldier on. In adulthood, this expectation is almost sadistic. If you don't smile through the "Big C" (like cancer is a character on Sesame Street), you're simply not made of stern-enough stuff. You are not enough of a warrior. And it's your fault for not keeping that chin up. Positive thinking is all that everyone is talking about, even when things look kind of negative. And yes, one's outlook on life cannot alleviate physical symptoms, but it has been shown to correlate with one's subjective evaluation of how they are feeling.

So far so good, right? Well, yes, except that, sometimes, you cannot and will not smile or think positively. As author Barbara Ehrenreich discovered when diagnosed with breast cancer, patient forums were not very receptive to her accounts of how she felt, which wasn't always all rosy-tinted. In her book *Bright-Sided: How Positive Thinking is Undermining America*, Ehrenreich points out that positive seeking has become somewhat of a cultural obsession. We judge negative feelings harshly, putting all too much faith in the nasty mirror image of positive thinking – the belief that negative thoughts breed negative outcomes.

In fact, would you be surprised to learn that new research shows that experiencing and accepting anger and sadness are vital to our mental health? According to Adler and Hershfield (2012), taking the good and the bad together "may detoxify" the bad experiences, allowing you to make meaning out of them in a way that supports psychological well-being.

So here's the bottom line: **allowing negative feelings some designated 'airtime' will actually help prevent you from getting consumed by them, counterintuitive though it may seem.**

EXERCISE

Write yourself a permission slip to mope in your journal. Include where, when and for how long you're going to feel the negative emotions—sadness, depression, frustration, anger, rage, or even hatred. You can choose to allow twenty minutes after dinner when alone and away from breakable dishes and there's no appetite to lose anymore. You can choose to do something or sit down and do nothing. Set the timer and like an exercise workout do a cool-down workout mental when you're done and carry on with your evening.

TIPS

Tip 1: If you choose to do it on a slip of paper be sure to upload a picture of your official permission slip here!

Tip 2: Respect the permission slip! When the time comes for you to mope, let the emotion come, feel it, and know that it's alright.

Tip 3: Learn to address each emotion as it comes. Check out our Declutter Your Mind course.

Tip 4: Your negative feelings are equally a part of you as your positive feelings. Check out our Cultivating Authenticity course to help you get acquainted with all your feelings.

DRIVING THE MESSAGE HOME

This extended clip of Disney's animated film, Inside Out, helps shed light on our core emotions, and how they influence us on a daily basis. Anger, fear, joy, sadness, and shame are just some of the many feelings we have. And yet, how often do we allow ourselves time to really experience our feelings in their entirety? We have so many emotions that have been 'exiled.' Part of emotional management means identifying our feelings, and feeling them, regardless of how challenging they are. After all, Joy mucks everything up by ignoring Sadness' role in Riley's brain. So take a moment to enjoy this animated film of the underpinnings of our brain. And then, take some time to mope.

Check out some clips from Disney's 2015 movie Inside Out on YouTube or plan a fun night of popcorn and relaxation and watch the full movie for an entertaining approach on the emotions that live in all of us!

8 Tips for days when emotional management is not gonna happen

When you're ill, you will probably have good days and bad days. Days when you are emotionally coping and days when you are totally not. Well, this list is geared to help you get through those bad ones.

1. Focus on the good days. Remember they are just around the corner and will be back very soon. Even during a relapse, you can have good days. Make the best of them when they come around, and when they don't, remember that they'll be back soon!
2. Have a plan for the not-so-good days. Imagine these days as a day off from work. Read, rest, have a cup of hot cocoa. Try not to feel guilty for doing nothing. You're entitled to this – you're sick! Prepare the books you can read (something light), a favorite sitcom, and maybe some easy listening too.
3. Allow for some occasional self-pity. If you're having a really bad day, allow yourself time to wallow and cry. Use this time to get out all of your frustrations, over your disease and your life. Grow from there.
4. Write. Having a journal where you can express how bad you are feeling on the bad days provides a safe container for you and your feelings.
5. Rest. Make sure you rest on the good days. I know it sounds hard, but your body with thank you for it. So will your mind.

Have any other ideas?

6. ____

7. ____

8. ____

It's hard to accept negative emotions around my illness because:

When it comes to accepting emotions, the positive ones always seem to vibe better than the negative ones. And yet, both equally impact our medical condition. What are some of the obstacles that stand in your way of embracing your negative emotions?

1. I'm afraid the negative emotions will consume me.

2. I don't have any negative feelings toward my illness.

3. I don't want others to think I'm depressed/anxious/anything else negative.

4. Negative emotions get in the way of me achieving my management goals for my actual medical condition.

5. Negative emotions are too unstructured and unpredictable for me.

Add your own:

6. ____

The time moping about my illness was a great idea

Sometimes there's no room for a stiff-upper-lip, and you just have to mope it out until you can feel better. Share with the community a time you needed to mope in order to feel better, and maybe inspire others to engage in a bit of well-timed moping.

Take some time brainstorming in your journal about your experience with managing your illness, and then share your story with the Buddy and Soul community! Direct message us YOUR story @Buddy_N_Soul on Instagram and be anonymously featured for a chance to **win a Buddy&Soul three month free membership**. Or post a picture and tag us on Instagram and Twitter @Buddy_N_Soul, using the **#BuddynSoulMedSupport**. By sharing with us on social media, not only can you help others with their personal journeys, you can read about those facing similar challenges.

My strongest feelings as I manage my illness are:

Part of emotionally managing your illness is identifying all the emotions you are feeling, even those you are experiencing simultaneously. Here are what are known as the core emotions. How much do you experience each of them?

1. **Happy.** I feel so at peace that I'm making an effort, even if it's not always smooth sailing.
2. **Sad.** This emotional management is making me realize how little control I have over everything.
3. **Angry.** I hate being sick, and I hate everything that reminds me of it!
4. **Afraid.** If I have to emotionally manage my medical condition… does that mean I'm really ill? This isn't just going away?
5. **Ashamed.** What kind of weak, sad, pathetic person needs help to keep their emotions in check? I'm not a moody teenager!
6. **Guilty.** This condition is taking such a toll on my family and friends, but only now am I realizing just how much.

Add your own:

7. ____

8. ____

9. ____

Strategy 6: Keep a full tank

When ill, a lot of our energy goes into dealing with lifestyle changes and maintenance (yes, yes, exercise and nutrition), measurements, keeping up with medication, stressing, and trying to feel better. Unfortunately, not too much fuel is left to drive you home, emotionally.

And as they say – something's gotta give. It's either your self-care, or your happiness. Not to mention your work, studies, or relationships. This is where the buck stops, though.

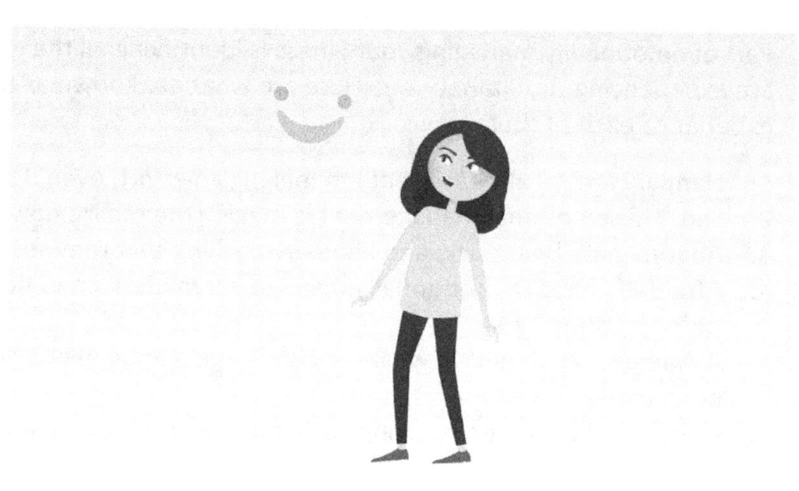

A friend of mine, a university department chair who developed a rare form of lymphoma, says it changed the way he communicates with colleagues, students and employees. "Before the disease," he says, "when someone entered my office, we would schmooze for an hour before getting to whatever they came to discuss. Now, when someone enters my office, I do not want to spend (or waste!) that hour. Instead I say 'state your intention'."

Cut to the chase. Energy efficient. Saving your resources for what matters.

Although "energy-efficiency" has as many faces as there are people managing illnesses out there, it's crucial to find out what expands or depletes your personal energy tank. Don't worry about feeling selfish. Your first duty at this time (and, really, at any time) is to yourself. As they say on the plane, put your oxygen mask on first, and then help others. You are the boss here – the only one who can manage your medical condition.

EXERCISE

Step 1: **Take this short survey:**

Leaving illness aside, what would make me feel pampered?

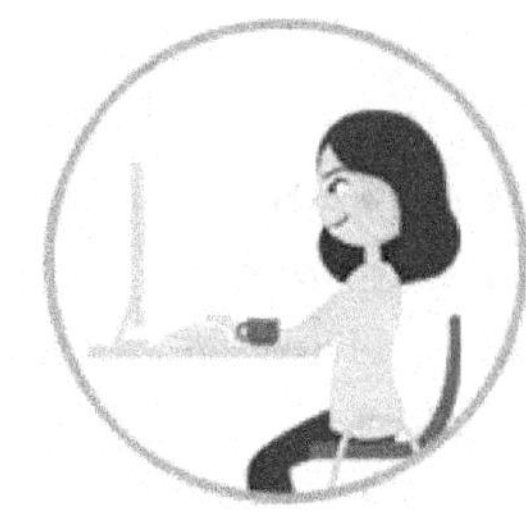

1. Focusing my attention outside of me by helping others.
2. Doing something fun and adventurous, like riding a rollercoaster.
3. Taking care of something that's been hanging over me, like my diet.
4. Taking care of my appearance.
5. Organizing my space so it's neat and clean.
6. Going out, or watching a movie.

Step 2: Keeping in mind what you rated highest in the survey in step 1**, write down one thing you are going to do this week that will fill your mental energy tank.** For example – if you marked 'Focusing on me, and me alone,' and a new book and take-out is your thing, take the time to do it properly.

TIPS

Tip 1: Now that you have an idea of where to start, and what you need to do to replenish your emotional energy, make it a priority to repeat and cherish these things. Take our Priorities Reboot course to help you.

Tip 2: Practicing this action does not mean you are selfish. It means you are performing your duty of taking good care of yourself.

Tip 3: Try to think of your day as a treasure hunt, looking for those great moments that replenish you and actually savoring them.

Tip 4: For more on upping your energy levels be sure to check out our Willpower 101 course.

DRIVING HOME THE MESSAGE

This session might help you deepen your motivation surrounding managing your illness. This involves understanding the value of saying No. Saying "no" is not only saying no. Rather, it's utilizing the power of no in order to grow. What do I mean? When we're younger our parents act as our yes/no conscience. However, when we get older we need to become our own conscience. We need to learn for ourselves when we should say yes, and when we should say no. It's not only about saying yes/no, it's about knowing when to say yes/no.

Noted entrepreneur and presentation expert Kenny Nguyen passionately speaks about the power inherent in saying "no." The CEO of Big Fish Presentations, Kenny speaks about how "no" has affected him personally and professionally, but more importantly, how it can prepare one for the perfect time to say yes. The word no is a way to protect us. Especially during this time of illness where we are simply unable to say yes all the time. So let's delve into the power of no, and learn for ourselves, when should we say yes, and when should we say no.

Watch 'The Art of Saying No' presented by Kenny Nguyen at TEDxLSU on YouTube.

6 Tips to fill you with energy

Even when you know where you want to be—filled with energy—it's hard to make it happen. Easier said than done, and all that. Here are some tips to help you fill your energy tank, so you don't get left hangin'.

(Plus: Check out our <u>Willpower 101 course</u> 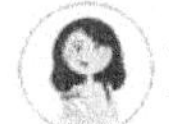)

1. When you find something that works for you, stick with it. No need to reinvent the wheel if you already know what works for you.

2. Keeping that in mind, don't be afraid to change your 'energy filler' if you've found that it's grown stale. Don't sit down to watch an episode of your favorite show if you no longer enjoy it!

3. When looking for something to refill your energy tanks, try and pick something manageable. A bout at a theme park always works for me, but the nearest one is a two-hour drive away... Not exactly practical for when I need a boost during a break at work.

Add your own!

4. ____

5. ____

6. ____

It's selfish to make this disease even more about me.

When people say "take the time for you" it sounds nice, but doesn't it really just boil down to being selfish? And if everyone did that, wouldn't the world economy basically collapse, or something like that? I don't want to be part of the selfish crowd.

For:

1. By definition, yes. It's selfish to make everything revolve around me.
2. I'm always talking about my dietary needs, meds, fears… And that's legitimate. Adding to that a little more selfishness? It's a bit much.
3. I have responsibilities to my job and family, and putting myself first necessarily means putting one of those things second. I'm just not prepared to be that person.

Add your own argument:

4. ____

Against:

1. Selfish doesn't have to be "mean". It could also be construed as selfish to take a bathroom break instead of just soldiering through 8 hours at the office. But you know what? Sometimes you have to be a bit "selfish" to remain sane.
2. You don't have to share this with anyone, if you're feeling self-conscious about the attention you're getting. But take the time to do something small for yourself, so you have the mental energy to continue with your day.
3. If you don't put yourself first, no one else will. And it will make you a better *everything* if you take the time to really care for your own needs, too.

Add your own argument:

4. ____

How having some fun helped me manage my illness

Instinctively, it doesn't seem like the best time for fun, but a spot of levity and shenanigans are sometimes just what's needed in order to effectively manage your illness, emotionally. Share with the community how you have fun in order to ease some of the emotional weight that comes with illness.

Take some time brainstorming in your journal about your experience with managing your illness, and then share your story with the Buddy and Soul community! Tag us on Instagram and Twitter @Buddy_N_Soul, using the **#BuddynSoulMedSupport**. Also direct message us YOUR story @Buddy_N_Soul on Instagram and be anonymously featured for a chance to **win a Buddy&Soul three month free membership**. By sharing with us on social media, not only can you help others with their personal journeys, you can read about those facing similar challenges.

4 Guilt-free reminders to say no as you manage your illness

We all know that saying yes to everything and everyone turns us into zombies. And yet, saying no can be so challenging! Here are some great, guilt-free reminders that will help you say no when you need to.

(Plus: Check out our Priorities Reboot course 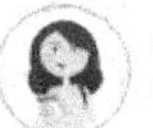)

1. The more you say no to the things you don't want to do, the more you will be able to say yes to the things you want to do.
2. It's better to say no and feel uncomfortable now than say yes and be resentful for the rest of your life.
3. Saying no builds character.
4. "No" is a protective shield to help you keep your energy up.

Accepting your sadness and making sure you're running on a full tank of emotional energy are necessary steps to emotionally managing your illness. Now it's time to look up, and see about actively finding positivity in your every-day life. Even on bleak days, positive moments are there, and it's our task to notice and experience them. It can be the difference between allowing your medical condition to live your life, as opposed to living your life with a medical condition.

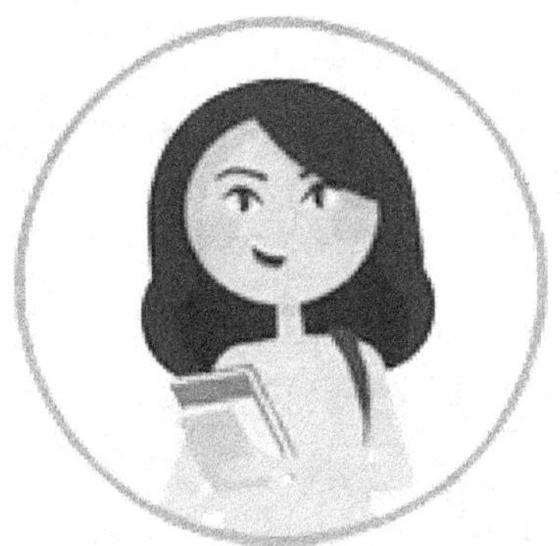

(Plus: Check out our Create a Pleasant Reality course 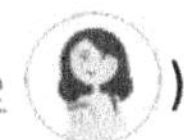)

Even at a time like this, you can feel happy. Your personal catalyst can be anything from taking time to enjoy a favorite activity with your child, watching a re-run of Sex and the City (shoe fetish notwithstanding), some chocolate, sunshine, the nurse smiled at me, they served meatloaf for lunch, you name it. Don't consider these real-happy moments as trivial, and don't dismiss them as being unrelated to the battle you're fighting – embrace them and try to enhance their presence in your life as a means of counterbalancing the unavoidable negatives. Some days will be blurs of gray, but that doesn't have to be the only color on your canvas. If you can find some splashes of color in unexpected places, it can turn your whole day around.

Research shows that positive emotions can help people in negative situations; when you are stuck in negative feelings or thoughts, such as grief, pessimism or isolation, encouraging (or even manufacturing) positive emotions will help you to take positive action. In addition, increasing happiness can help reduce the pain from a negative life event.

We aren't trying to say you should only be happy (after all, we did make time to mope). **Yet just like you made space for your negative feelings, now it's time to make space for the positive emotions as well.**

EXERCISE

List 3 positive things that happened to you today, no matter how small
(*someone left me just enough milk for a cup of coffee; I had all WALK signals on my daily walk; I caught a hilarious segment on the Tonight Show*).

Can't think of 3? Try harder! Think of small things that added just a splash of color to your day.

TIPS

Tip 1: Make a habit of finding these things as they occur, and being grateful for them. Check out our Habit Workshop course for more on habit formation.

Tip 2: Try to use laughter as a healing tool too! Although it may seem counter-intuitive, now is when you need a good laugh more than ever.

Tip 3: Use your Buddy&Soul journal to keep a running list of the daily sources of happiness you find.

DRIVING THE MESSAGE HOME

Thank you for joining us for this next happy session. Nobody wakes up every morning and thinks, how can we suffer today? That might be a clear indicator that we humans have a deep innate desire for meaning and happiness. And yet how can we attain happiness? What is happiness, and how can we all get some? Biochemist turned Buddhist monk Matthieu Ricard says we can train our minds in habits of well-being, to generate a true sense of serenity and fulfillment. In his humble opinion, happiness, or well-being, comes from the establishment of healthy habits.

And how can we tap into the 'well-being' state of mind? Through mindfulness and brain plasticity and experiencing happiness as you emotionally manage your illness is crucial. It will help provide you with the energy you need to carry on and find meaning in your life. This Ted Talk will help you think about how you can use healthy habits to train your mind to experience a lot more happiness in your life.

(Plus: Check out our Mindfulness for Beginners and Habit Workshop courses 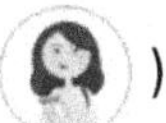)

Watch 'The Habits of Happiness' presented by Matthieu Ricard on YouTube.

Laugh? When my body is failing me?

Laughter is the way your body reacts when the completely unexpected happens. It is usually expressed when a person is having an absolute blast. Illness is so not that. How can I think about laughing at a time like this? Or is it really a time like this that laughter can help me the most?

For:

1. I need to be focused on what the doctors are saying, on my medication regiment and other assorted serious matters. This is no time for laughing.
2. Laughing is for kids. We adults need to take life more seriously.
3. I barely have enough air to breathe, let alone to laugh.
4. With all that's going on, I can't think of a single thing that's funny these days.
5. If I laugh, the medical staff and other caregivers won't take me seriously.

Add your own argument:

6. ____

Against:

1. Laughing makes us feel better. Look at toddlers they laugh hundreds of times a day, and they're happy most of the time. We adults laugh about 15 times a day, no wonder we give in to stress so easily.
2. Laughing gets the diaphragm moving and this plays a vital part in moving blood around the body, which in turn, can aid the healing process.
3. Laughter also helps in oxygenating the body by boosting the respiratory system.
4. Laughing will lighten you up and relax you. It can help you clear your head so you can remember all those instructions more easily.
5. Laughter can break the tension with those around you, caregivers, family, friends.
6. I don't lose anything by laughing, so I'd rather do that than mope.

Add your own argument:

7. ____

9 Little happiness boosters

When you're sick and you feel like life just sucks, it's nice to have some things that can really cheer you up. Here are some ideas but I'm sure you can think of many more!

(Plus: Check out our Create a Pleasant Reality Course 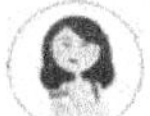)

1. Taking a long, luxurious bath. You can do it at home, and it's the type of pampering you don't usually make time for.

 2. A bought cup of coffee. It's so much cheaper to just pour yourself a cup at home but sometimes going out for something so simple can make a big difference.

 3. When's the last time you laughed and couldn't stop? Grab a friend and head to the movie theater to see a comedy. Or even find one you want to see and watch it at home.

 4. Like gardening? Head to your local nursery and pick up a new plant. And if you're not the greatest of gardeners, just buy yourself some bright, fragrant flowers. You're worth it!

5. Speaking of fragrant things – buy a new, fancy shower gel or lotion.

6. Take the day off and go on a mini vacation. Explore some area where you've never been. A new perspective can feel really good.

Add your own:

7. ____

8.____

9. ____

When I finally let myself be happy

For a long time, it felt as though if I worried enough, that was doing my part in managing this illness. As though it would prove to the universe that I was taking it seriously. But then something happened and I accidentally let myself be happy despite my illness, and it changed how I saw everything. When did you finally allow yourself to be happy, despite your better judgement?

Direct message us YOUR story @Buddy_N_Soul on Instagram and be anonymously featured for a chance to **win a Buddy&Soul three month free membership**. Share the wisdom!

Happiness when I'm sick? Forget about it!

There's something about the sick person mentality that means being miserable all the time. It's the way of the world. I can try to challenge that, but it won't work, not really.

(Plus: Check out our Cultivating Authenticity course 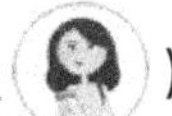)

For:

1. I'm so sick of people trying to sugarcoat illness. It sucks.   In every way.
2. If I'm happy when I'm sick then people may think I'm happy about being sick. I definitely don't want to give off that impression!
3. Happiness means accepting what's going on with me right now. There's no way I'm going to accept my illness.
4. What's happy about being sick, may I ask you?
5. When I give off the impression that I'm dealing and coping and managing, people assume I'm fine and strong and capable, and don't offer me help or sympathy. And you know what? I'm sick of being capable. I want to be weak and to fall apart. I deserve it.

Add your own argument:

6. ____

Against:

1. Being physically sick doesn't mean being emotionally sick. You can be sick and happy. And also be healthy and unhappy.
2. Why do happiness and illness have to be opposites?
3. Being ill takes away so much of myself. I'm not going to let it take away my happiness too.
4. My soul and spirit will never be harmed by my illness.
5. Not to sound preachy but I'm gaining a lot of positive things from being sick. For example, I've never been so grateful in my life for the simple every day pleasures I now experience in totality.
6. Being happy during illness is actually shown to alter your physical health.

Add your own argument:

7. ____

<u>Strategy 8: Reframe and rename your difficulties</u>

According to the theory of narrative identity, beginning in adolescence, individuals start constructing their 'story', which includes their reconstructed past, the perceived present and their anticipated future. Meaning they start forming a story, weaving together all the interpretations of past experiences, what is going on with them now, and what they want their future to be like. This dynamic is always at work in the back of your mind.

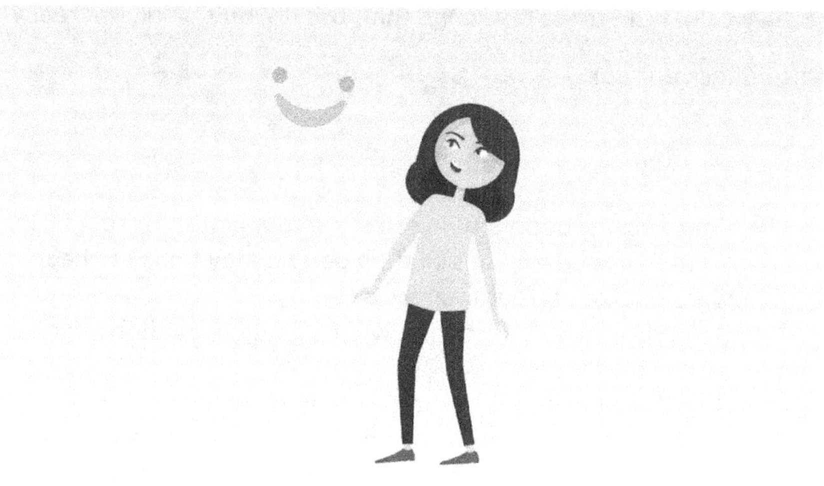

I have a friend who, in her adolescent years, was happily classified as a religiously healthy-eater. Whole wheat *anything*, huge green salads, and interesting new grains whenever she could find them. When she was diagnosed with Crohn's, however, the carpet was pulled from under her: someone telling her to avoid the foods that she not only loved, but that she was always told were healthiest. It was a nightmare. It was like someone who took everything she was and clicked "undo", leaving her unsure of who she was. For a few weeks, her story was how miserable she was, how she couldn't enjoy anything, how food had lost its fun...

But then, her story changed. It became how she'd become like an 18th century noblewoman, insisting on white bread, rice and couscous. By reframing her current status (no longer able to eat what she wanted), and renaming her current status (nobility), she had effectively changed her reality. Of course, if a magical cure became available tomorrow she'd happily go back to her previous eating habits... But until then, **why live with a sad story when you can tell a happy one?**

EXERCISE

In your journal, **identify areas in your life that get you down.** It can be the dietary restrictions, the medical regime that makes it hard to travel, or the cloud of stigma that you feel floats over you along with the word "disease". Outline briefly what distresses you about your chosen area(s).

Then, **try offering a different name for how you're feeling and finding a new 'wrapping' for it that allows you to tell the same facts in a more positive tone.** For example, instead of focusing on the new foods your body needs, perhaps reframe them as medicine and thus non-negotiable.

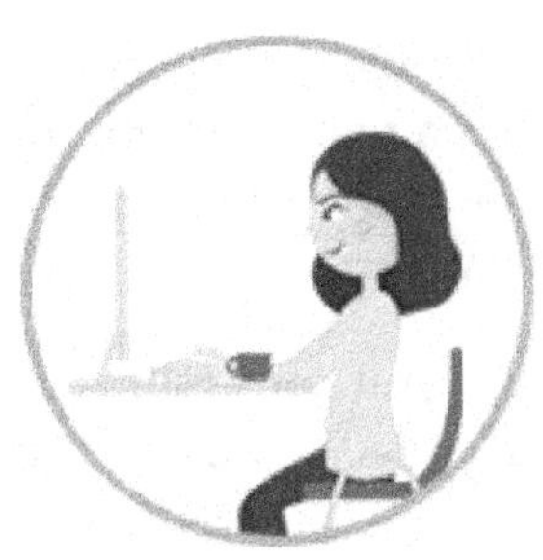

TIPS

Tip 1: When you're done the session, this action, like all actions, will be available in your journal, so revisit it whenever you're feeling blue about your situation.

Tip 2: No element is too large or too small to reframe, so keep going until you have an overall story you're happy with.

Tip 3: Memorize the new story, until it's second nature to you. You'll be surprised how strange the old story sounds after even a few days!

Tip 4: Check out our Everyday Reframing course 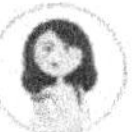 for more on rewriting your life's script.

Tip 5: If it's hard, try thinking of how you would describe your condition to someone who is gravely ill (and worse off than you).

Tip 6: Check out our Defining Your Identity course 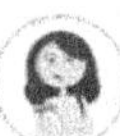 for tools on defining who you are with your illness.

DRIVING THE MESSAGE HOME

Many people roll their eyes when they hear someone say, "98 years *young*". Okay, we get you're trying to make a point about age and playfulness and mental youth, but 98 is old, no matter how you cut it. But the truth of the matter is, somethings *do* change when you make an effort to frame them differently.

The way you name something is the way you perceive it, and eventually it becomes the only truth you can see. Are your cloths old or vintage? Is your home cramped or quaint? As Rory Sutherland explains in this exceptional TED Talk, perspective is everything, and unlike so many things in life, this is something we have the power to control.

Watch 'Perspective is Everything' presented by Rory Sutherland on YouTube.

8 More hopeful reframes for your illness

Reframing is great… But you can only truly comprehend just how awesome the reframe is when you're struggling with an illness.

(Plus: Check out our Everyday Reframing course 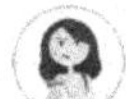)

1. You're discovering strengths you never knew you had.
2. You get a chance to truly focus on you and your health.
3. You've been given the ability to assess your life until now. Maybe it's time for a change and without this time to stop and think, you never would have realized it.
   (Plus: Check out our Tackling Change course)
4. Look how many people all around you love you and want to help. Before your illness you never would have had a chance to witness this outpouring of love.
5. When your illness forces you to lay low, you finally get a chance to let your body catch up on its much-needed rest.

Add your own:

6. ____

7. ____

8. ____

What helps you reframe your illness?

It's been proven that reframing works, but for a subject as laden as chronic illness it might be a bit harder to access all the benefits of reframing. Which of the following aspects did you find most useful when reframing your disease difficulties?
(Plus: Check out our Everyday Reframing course).

1. Finding a different name for something I was experiencing. Titles are everything.
2. Separating the feelings from the facts. I can work with facts.
3. Not going at it immediately, but giving myself time to come to terms with my current story before trying to implement a new one.
4. Repetition. I found that in order to believe the new story, I had to say it lots of times in a row.
5. Starting small and working my way up to larger reframes.

Add your own:

6. ____

7. ____

8. ____

The reframe that changed my whole illness experience

Nothing can change being ill, but there are ways to see the illness as something more than wholly negative. Share with the community what reframe, large or small, helped you change your experience, and perhaps you can inspire others to reframe, as well.

Take some time brainstorming in your journal about your experience with your medical condition, and then share your story with the Buddy and Soul community! Direct message us YOUR story @Buddy_N_Soul on Instagram and be anonymously featured for a chance to **win a Buddy&Soul three month free membership**. Share the wisdom! You can also tag us on Instagram and Twitter @Buddy_N_Soul, using the **#BuddynSoulMedSupport**. By sharing with us on social media, not only can you help others with their personal journeys, you can read about those facing similar challenges.

The unlikely silver lining I discovered with my illness

While there is no question that being ill really, really, stinks, there are sometimes some silver linings that only we can see. What were some of the unlikely silver linings that came with the territory of being ill, for you?

Take some time brainstorming in your journal about your experience with your medical condition, and then share your story with the Buddy and Soul community! Tag us on Instagram and Twitter @Buddy_N_Soul, using the **#BuddynSoulMedSupport**. By sharing with us on social media, not only can you help others with their personal journeys, you can read about those facing similar challenges.

<u>Strategy 9: Give to others</u>

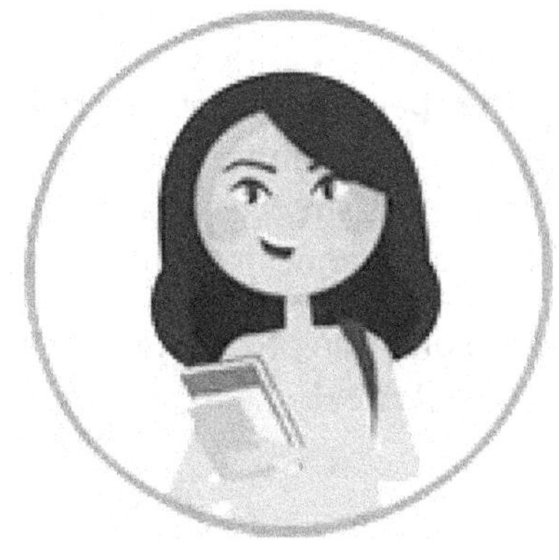

You might think it's ridiculous, or just wrong. You're sick; you're not feeling well. You might be frightened. And here we are asking you to *give*? Well, yes. That's exactly what we are advocating. Giving is a way to feel good about yourself and to feel vibrantly needed. **At a time when you might be leaning on others for support – emotional and other – it is important to also feel that others can lean on you, or at least cherish something that you can give.** Additionally, studies demonstrate that giving to others, whether it is your time or money, creates more happiness than when giving to oneself (Mogilner & Norton, 2016; Pholphirul, 2014).

What can you give, you wonder? Don't think major investments! You know that box of macaroons your neighbor got you which is still sitting in your freezer because of the high sugar content? Offer one to your visiting niece, or to the nice man who brings you your mail at the office, or to the friend who came to visit and looks even more exhausted than you feel.

No macaroons? How about giving a kind word, a smile, or a compliment? Thank your friends, family, and doctors for taking care of you. Not just because they'll appreciate it, but rather because it will remind you of your own worth and of your ability to give. Tell one of your visitors how much you appreciate them coming over. Or tell someone who called you that she made you happy. This will also help change your perspective and get you to focus on what you have.

In his book *The Positive Principle Today*, Dr. Norman Vincent Peal, a progenitor of the theory of "positive thinking" claims that "…when you become detached mentally from yourself and concentrate on helping people with *their* difficulties, it is a fact that you will be able to cope with your own more effectively. Somehow, the act of self-giving is a personal power-releasing factor" (2007, p. 168).

This is not a lone voice on the power of giving, either. In their book *Why Good Things Happen to Good People*, Dr. Stephen Post, a professor of preventative medicine at Stony Brook University, and writer Jill Neimark, bring scientific research that proves that the power of giving is so potent that it increases health benefits in people with chronic illness.

EXERCISE

Use the space in our journal to identify ways or things that you could give (a hug, a smile, a penny, a hand in carrying groceries, holding the door). It can be something as small as a kind word you would have otherwise neglected to say or as large as a random act of kindness to a stranger.

Choose one thing from your list and commit to giving at least *some*thing to *some*one today!

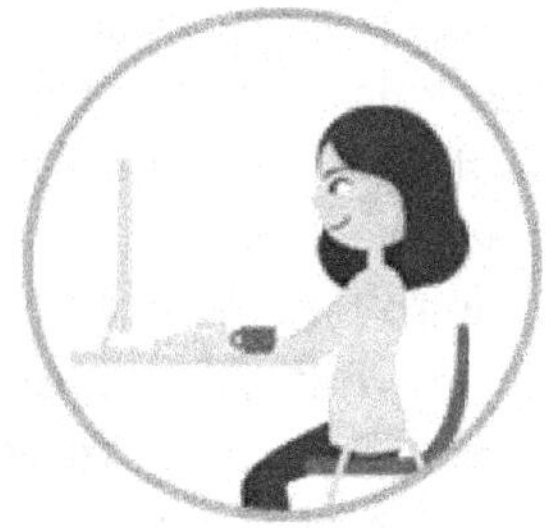

TIPS

Tip 1: No act of giving is too small. You might be surprised at how happy you'll make the other person with even just a smile or a kind word.

Tip 2: Make giving to others a priority in your life. Check out our Priorities Reboot course. 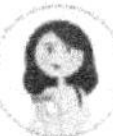

DRIVING THE MESSAGE HOME

We think you'll enjoy the next clip, it's a recipe for the Good Life (capital letters) with data.

What keeps us happy and healthy as we go through life? If you think it's fame and money, you're not alone – but, according to psychiatrist Robert Waldinger, you're mistaken. As the director of a 75-year study on adult development, Waldinger has unprecedented access to data on happiness and satisfaction. In this talk, he shares three important lessons learned from the study as well as some practical, old-as-the-hills wisdom on how to build a fulfilling, long life. Although I won't spill the punch line, all three of these important lessons deliver one universal message: good relationships keep us healthier and happier. So, take some time to invest in your relationships and to give to others. By leaning in to your relationships you are betting both your body and your mind.

Watch 'What Makes a Good Life? Lessons from the Longest Study on Happiness' presented by Robert Waldinger on YouTube.

What deters you from giving while you're managing illness?

As someone with an illness, giving can be so beneficial. And yet, sometimes you're just not in the mood. What holds you back from giving as a way to help you emotionally manage your illness?

1. I'm too tired.
2. I don't have the physical capability to give to someone.
3. I don't have the emotional capability to give to someone.
4. Procrastination. I'm always thinking, tomorrow I'll give.
5. I don't know anybody I'd actually want to give to.

Add your own:

6. ____

7. ____

8. ____

6 Giving hacks for self-conscious types

Giving is a great way to help you and the people you are giving to feel great! However, for the self-conscious, giving can be really challenging. How can you give when you are concerned that people will be judging you? Here are some great tips to help you jumpstart your giving now.

1. Start small. Share a cookie with a friend, smile at your neighbor walking by, give your sad friend a hug. These little acts of giving are incredibly meaningful and won't give you a 'what will other people think complex.'
2. Give in private. There's lots of giving that can be done in the privacy of your own home, free from the watchful eyes of family and friends.
3. Go someplace new. There's nothing like being in a new place with new people that will give you the confidence to try giving.

Any other ideas?

4. ____

5. ____

6. ____

Why giving was my greatest teacher

Paradoxically, giving to someone else can actually help you more than you think. Read below to get inspired by how others gave, and received in return, and share your own story with the community.

Direct message us YOUR story @Buddy_N_Soul on Instagram and be anonymously featured for a chance to **win a Buddy&Soul three month free membership**. Share the wisdom!

How my medical condition taught me the value of relationships

Like many people, I took relationships for granted until my medical condition forced me to look some of them in the eye. I suddenly saw my relationships, even the most casual ones, in a new light. Here's how.

Strategy 10: I have a dream

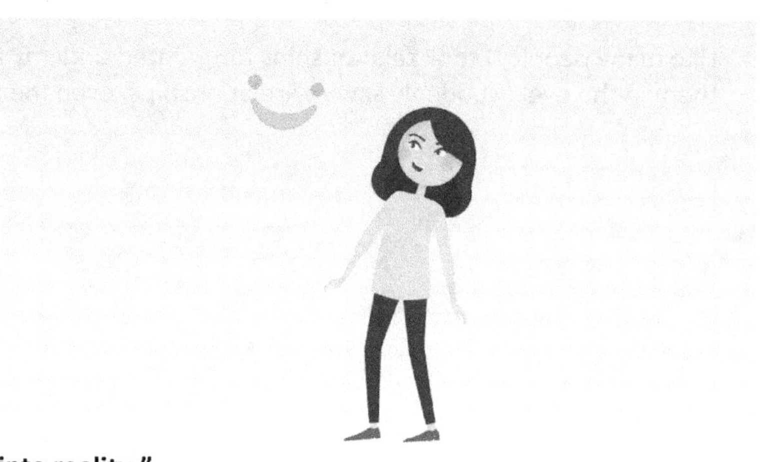

Visualization is a very powerful tool. It allows our mind to explore and familiarize itself with ideas, concepts and realities (currently) out of reach. It can also offer a respite from our current reality, and when where we are is sick and aching, that's a blessed thing. An image and a dream can be something you aspire to, even if they seem very far at the moment. **As Jonas Salk so wisely put it, "Hope lies in dreams, in imagination, and in the courage of those who dare to make dreams into reality."**

(Plus: Check out our Achieve Your Goals course 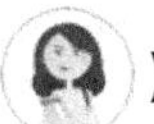)

So start mobilizing your dreams today. Go for it! It can be one tiny step at a time.

Something like writing about your childhood on a Wisconsin farm, embroidering the Mona Lisa, attending a Billy Joel concert in Madison Square Garden, starting a local exhibition of watercolors, or arranging a family reunion that brings together people from four continents.

A dream deserves time to soak in both when you're forming it and when you're fulfilling the dream. While working on healing from, or living with, an illness can keep your hands full, having a dream will give you something to look forward to and a purpose to follow. Some days the dream may take a back seat, but on others you may find that immersing yourself in something other than your illness provides a much-needed relief.

While healing from surgery and intensive chemo and radiation, author and public speaker Michele Cushatt launched her book *Undone: Making Peace with an Imperfect Life*. She writes in her blog about how it took seven years to write and two years to edit. When it finally launched, it was on the worst day possible. And yet it was the best day possible.

When working with dreams, let go of control and instead embrace the unknown. Any dream you build may not have the timetable you want and may not go exactly according to your plan. But this added sense of purpose that is entirely *yours* will help renew your sense of direction.

A dream will help you make your life about more than just the disease.

EXERCISE

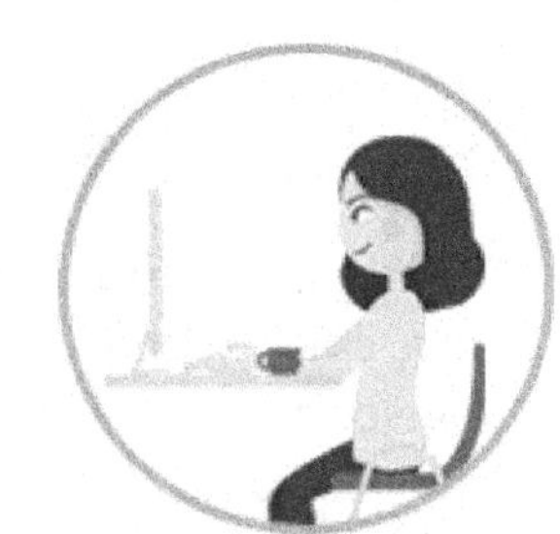

Step 1: **Use your journal to write freely about your life dreams.** What would give you a sense of joy, meaning, and purpose beyond the daily realities of managing your condition?

Step 2: **Choose one of your dreams and upload an image to Instagram that represents what it means you** (it can be abstract if you're not ready to share your dream quite yet). You can tag us on Instagram and Twitter @Buddy_N_Soul, using the **#BuddynSoulMedSupport**. By sharing with us on social media, not only can you help others with their personal journeys, you can read about those facing similar challenges. Revisit this image again and again, every time you feel a motivation landslide coming on.

TIPS

Tip 1: For bonus points, you can even start thinking about what steps you'll take to start mobilizing your dreams...

Tip 2: If you feel people around you may consider your dream silly, don't share. It'll be our little secret.

Tip 3: Some things are fun to dream about even if we have no intention of achieving them. Those dreams are sweet and valuable, too!

Tip 4: This could be a long-term dream, something to work towards and look forward to, or it could be a short-term, gotta-have-it-now, kind of dream that will simply brighten your day, week, month or year.

DRIVING THE MESSAGE HOME

Dreaming of the final session, here it is, we hope you gained much from this ten-part series.

What are your dreams? Better yet, what are your broken dreams? Dan Pallotta dreams of a time when we are as excited, curious and scientific about the development of our humanity as we are about the development of our technology. Pallota explains that we need to dream in more than one dimension; we need to not only dream for a better life in the future, but also to dream for a better life in the present. We need to dream about authentically and not only about productivity.

And what holds us back? We fear not being able to accomplish our dreams. However, to be human means to live with this fear. So let's transcend where we are now and take a step closer to accomplishing our dreams. In all dimensions.

Watch 'The Dream We Haven't Dared to Dream' presented by Dan Pallotta on YouTube.

How can I dream when I'm consumed with my illness?

Dreaming and positive thinking are all very nice. However, it's not going to change a very important fact. I have a disease!

(Plus: Check out our Achieve Your Goals course 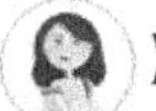)

For:

1. I need to focus on managing my illness on a daily basis, and not waste my time dreaming about some far-off place in the future
2. I like to focus on the concrete facts at hand, like this one: I have a disease.
3. What's the point of dreaming and imagining the future? My illness isn't simply going to evaporate one day with a wave of a wand.

Add your own argument:

4. ____

Against:

1. Dreaming is what will give me strength to physically and emotionally manage my illness daily.
2. Dreaming about finding happiness and stability with my illness is what will allow me to get there!
3. Without dreaming I have little motivation to persevere.

Add your own argument:

4. ____

What dreams helped you emotionally manage your illness?

I don't have to tell you that suffering from an illness is no fun. What dreams do you have that help you emotionally manage your illness?

1. I imagine who I was before I received my diagnosis and dream of returning to that me one day.
2. I fantasize about being on a deserted island without any hospital or doctors, surrounded by my loved ones and all the ice cream I could eat!
3. I dream about turning my story into a bestselling novel… and maybe a blockbuster movie after that!
4. Amazingly or not, I dream about getting back to the boring routine that I used to have.
5. For one whole day, I'd love being so immersed in something so much bigger than I am, that I don't even have time to remember my illness.

Add your own:

6. ____

7. ____

8. ____

The dream that allowed me to emotionally manage my illness

Sometimes, it seems that having something to hold on to, no matter how trivial or seemingly unimportant, is more important than medicine, and more of a motive to carry on than even our personal wellbeing. Read on to be inspired by the dreams that helped members of the community emotionally manage their illness.

The tiny dream I achieved, even with a medical condition

So many things get put on hold when you're ill, that it's important to stop and achieve whatever small dream you can. Because dreams are like hope; sometimes even just a tiny bit is enough. Share with the community the dreams you were able to achieve, and how it helped you emotionally manage your illness.

Take some time brainstorming in your journal about your experience with your medical condition, and then share your story with the Buddy and Soul community! Tag us on Instagram and Twitter @Buddy_N_Soul, using the **#BuddynSoulMedSupport**. You can also direct message us YOUR story @Buddy_N_Soul on Instagram and be anonymously featured for a chance to **win a Buddy&Soul three month free membership**. By sharing with us on social media, not only can you help others with their personal journeys, you can read about those facing similar challenges.

WHERE DO WE GO FROM HERE?

You've finished the Emotionally Manage Your Medical Conditions book, but you haven't finished the journey. It doesn't end, it just gets better. Revisit this book, carry its ideas with you. Check out BuddynSoul.com and the rest of our books for all we have to offer. Spread the word. And change your life for good.

Create a Pleasant Reality.

Whether you've found yourself struggling with depression or are just looking to make your day-to-day life more enjoyable, this book is for you. We've created this book as a multimedia tool for you to learn how to create a pleasant reality. You can do it. And we all need it.

<u>Goals you can achieve from reading 'Create a Pleasant Reality':</u>

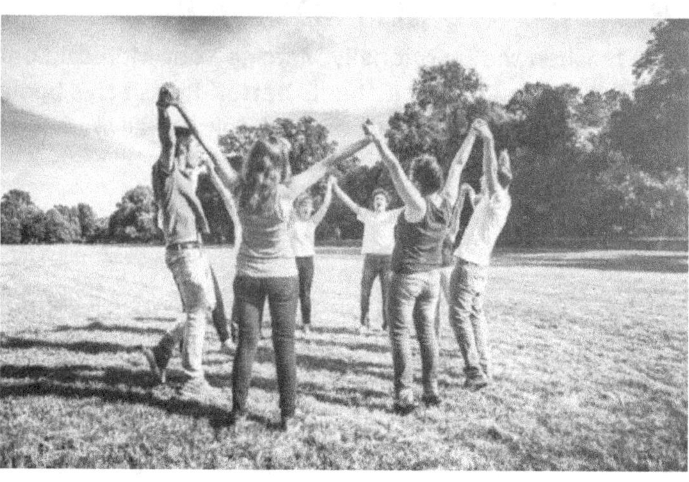

1. Understand what holds you back from enjoying life.
2. Learn tools to change the things you can and embrace the things you can't.
3. Tap into the power of ordinary moments to add joy and meaning to your life.

Manage your Medical Condition.

Being diagnosed with a medical
condition is just the start. It marks the
beginning of a journey into the
unknown. And, whether you like it or
not, on this journey, you are the captain
of that boat! Or at least, the co-captain,
alongside your physician. Because, let's
face it, there are very few situations in
which your involvement is not at all
required. Even by opening your mouth
to swallow a pill.

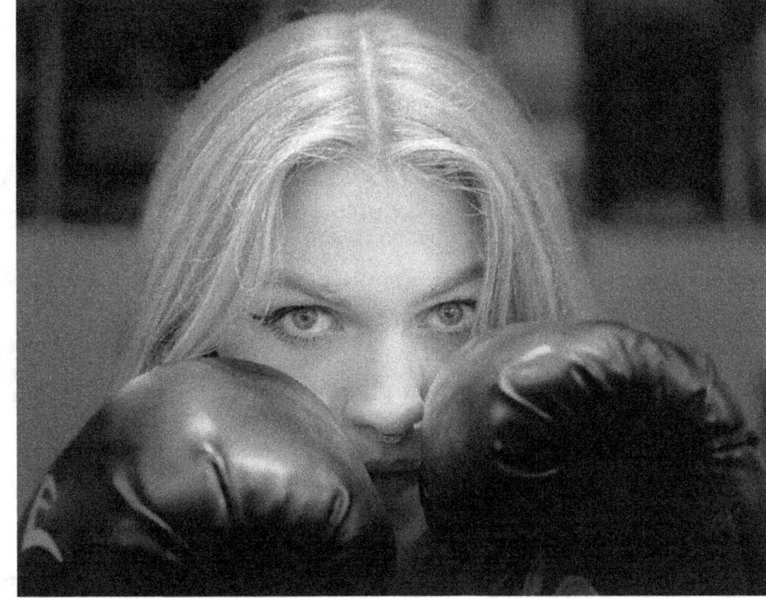

Goals you can achieve from reading
'Manage your Medical Condition':

1. Gain tools to actively manage your health.
2. Learn how to sort through and interpret medical information.
3. Assume responsibility for how you manage your medical condition.

Adhering to Your Medication.

Taking your medication is vital, especially when it comes to optimizing your long-term health. And yet, if you're taking this course, you know how hard it is to take your medication in a timely and efficient manner. And to do it all the time! This course offers you a fresh new look into adhering to your medication by exploring the cognitive, emotional, and behavioral elements that may be preventing you from improving your medication adherence, and your health outcomes.

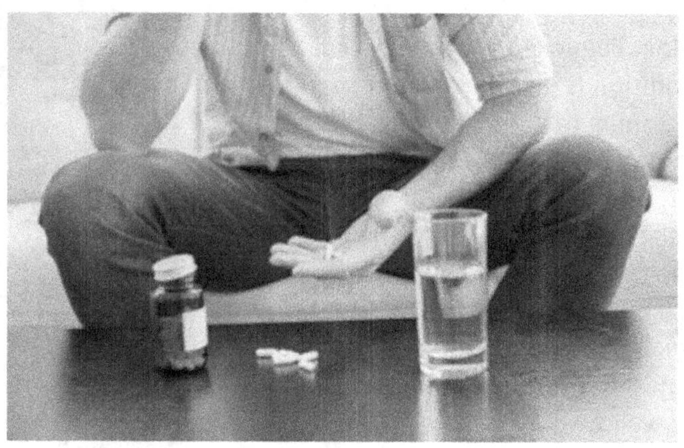

Goals you can achieve from reading 'Adhering to Your Medication':

1. Delve a little deeper into what may be holding you back from optimal adherence.
2. Learn practical tools to help ensure you take your meds as needed.
3. Assume responsibility for how you handle adherence to medication.

WANT TO LEARN MORE? CHECK THESE OUT!

MOVIES

Return to Me (2000)

Grace Briggs, a woman suffering from heart disease since the age of 14, is now in need of an immediate heart transplant to save her life. Grace ends up receiving the heart of Elizabeth Rueland who died in a car accident. A year after her transplant, Grace meets and falls in love with Elizabeth's widower Bob; at first unaware of the connection between them, what happens when Bob finds out that Grace holds Elizabeth's heart?

This movie is an excellent reminder that emotionally managing your medical condition can last long after the acute symptoms disappear, and that sometimes loved ones are the ones who need to manage the emotional fallout, as well.

Into the Wind (2010)

Based on a true story, 18-year-old Terry Fox had his leg amputated to prevent the spread of osteosarcoma (cancer of the bone). In order to raise money for cancer research he proposes the 'Marathon of Hope,' an individual Marathon in which Terry plans to run across Canada.

This is a movie about hope and the power of willpower and perseverance to help you accomplish your dreams.

MORE VIDEOS

Watch Shepherd's Powerful Story

Janine Shepherd was a cross-country skier training for the Olympics when a truck hit her during a training session. Here she tells the tale about the power of the human potential for recovery. Her powerful message: "You are not your body, and giving up old dreams can allow new ones to soar."

Watch Dr. Ochberg's fascinating talk

Ever wonder about the correlation between your mental and emotional health? Watch Dr. Frank Ochberg talk about the growing field of psychoneuroimmunology, or the study of the interactions between psychological processes and the nervous and immune systems of the human body.

BOOKS

Tuesdays with Morrie, by Mitch Albom

This book tells the tale of the author Mitch Albom and his relationship with his former college professor, Morrie Schwartz. Although twenty years had passed, Mitch felt the need to reconnect to his former prof., only to find him in the last months of his life. This inspirational and heartfelt book is based on the final meetings Mitch and Morrie had together in which the lessons on how to truly live are conveyed, and passed on to the next generation.

As you read the book, consider: does being ill necessarily mean losing hope?

The Diving Bell and the Butterfly: A Memoir of Life in Death, by Jean-Dominique Bauby

In 1995, Jean-Dominique Bauby, aged 44 was the editor-in chief of French *Elle*. He was known for his wit, style, and passionate way of living. However, a stroke to the brainstem left his entire body paralysed except for his left eye, which allowed him to see, and blink as a way of communicating to the world. This novel was dictated by blinking by Bauby, one letter at a time.

Bauby explores life and death via his left eye, and his story serves as a powerful reminder that a medical condition can bring your life to a screeching halt, but you nonetheless might be able to find a way forward.

GADGETS AND PRODUCTS

My Health, A Medical Records Journal - Kraft Hard Cover

This medical journal is a great way to get motivated to write about managing your medical condition. It provides prompts on every page to write about your symptoms, feelings, and doctors' recommendations.

Adulting notepad

This note pad will keep you on track while keeping your good spirits up as you "adult" your way through your medical career.

A great way to remind yourself to get things done without taking them too seriously, especially as you're emotionally managing an illness.